MW01120830

SEND SUICIDE PACKING

There's Something We Can
All Do to Help

Janet MacDonald

First Edition

youmattereveryday@gmail.com

ISBN: 978-1089474388

For Lisa. The bravest person I know.

Acknowledgements

Thank you to everyone who shared their personal stories and insights. I will be forever indebted. Thank you to those who made the writing of the book possible. Special thanks to Jamie, my personal editor, cheerleader and coach. I couldn't have done it without you. Thank you Kimberly, Lisa, April and Shamus for being supportive. Thank you to Genesis Davies of Upwork for using your literary finesse in a kind and encouraging manner and to Julia Bramer of Upwork for your superb formatting skills and business knowledge. Thank you to Infinite Sign from 99 Designs for understanding the importance of my book cover. Thank you to those that read the book and helped.

To anyone reading the book I would be honored to hear your comments. Please email: me at youmattereveryday@gmail.com.

Contents

1··WHY?

Introduction

When the call came from the police officer, I was ecstatic. They had found our 20-year-old daughter, Lisa, who had been lost in the woods for the past three hours. Then he told me there had been a very serious suicide attempt, which he described as "by a lethal means."

Luck was on her side, he exclaimed. Many aren't so lucky. She didn't have a change of heart, but luck did.

I couldn't believe it. How could my loving, talented daughter want to die? Why didn't she come to us for help? Why didn't we notice anything different?

This is what Lisa told us in the following days and years after her suicide attempt: "I didn't want to die; I just wanted this pain to stop. I couldn't figure out any other way to make the pain stop. I was convinced I was a burden on my family and friends, and they would be better off without me. When I would have the thought that I should tell someone what's going on, I also had the thought that no one could help, there wasn't any help, or it wouldn't make any difference. This was the only solution I could come up with. I had the continuing thought that it wasn't going to get any better. Things will never change. These thoughts had been around for a long time, maybe years. These thoughts in my head were very convincing. Maybe early on I knew the thoughts were ridiculous, but then there was a point where they were so believable. Having suicidal thoughts on and off for years, it starts to become the norm. My illness convinced me this was a way out. It started to comfort me, knowing the pain would finally stop. Besides, I thought, I am tired of putting my family through the highs and lows of my mental illness. If I was dead, they wouldn't have to worry about me anymore. These thoughts just wouldn't stop." How could this be? She was definitely not a burden to our family. We loved her above and beyond. If she asked for help, we would all be there for her – no rock unturned. We would not be better off without her; our lives would be never the same. How could she have spent six years having suicidal thoughts and not once shared with us? Where did these thoughts come from? How did this happen? We ponder the same questions when we mourn the lives of those that have died by suicide; Robin Williams, Kate Spade, Tim Bergling (Avicii), Anthony Bourdain, someone from our old high school, your friend's uncle, and beautiful youthful faces that appear in the obituary column of the morning newspaper requesting donations to the suicide crisis line. It's incomprehensible.

Jamie and I were high school sweethearts. We married after university and had some indulgent adventures before starting a family. Kimberly was the first born and was the pioneer of our family. She would have to experience all the firsts of growing up, both the good and the bad. She would be blazing a trail for the others to follow.

Lisa was the second, born three years later. She was full of adventure: nonstop play, and nonstop talk. She patented the phrase, "what do you want to do now?" She was always trying to keep pace with her older sister.

April arrived two years later. Not to be outdone by the older sisters, she was the self-taught whisperer for all animals in the house; dogs, cats, rabbits, gerbils, hamsters, and hermit crabs. Her room was the animal haven.

Shamus came last, but certainly not least. With three older sisters, he would acquire skills from an estrogen-infused household that would serve him well in life. Most days, he stayed out of active fire, methodically plotting his course.

These were busy times, but they were great times. The family calendar on the fridge looked like the logistical plan of air traffic control at a busy airport. Who's coming and who's going? There was hockey, soccer, drama, dance, girl guides, Tai Kwon Do, Beavers, and basketball. There was never a shortage of in-house entertainment.

Around the time Lisa turned fourteen, her mood changed. The happy go lucky, energy-infused child was changing. We hoped it was just part of the teenage years, but she didn't rebound. Not wanting to hang out with her friends as before. Staying in her room for long stretches of time. Hating school, which she had loved before. When it didn't pass, we took her to the doctor. What followed was six years of working through a maze of doctors, therapists, and medications. She was diagnosed with a mental illness. There were lots of ups and downs.

Lisa had just returned home in April after spending the school year away at Community College four hours away. Jamie and I had struggled with the decision to let her go away to school, which she wanted to do. We breathed a sigh of relief when she arrived back home for the summer. There had been some challenges in the school year, and toward the end of the year she started seeing a new therapist. We thought things were looking up. We certainly didn't see her suicide attempt coming.

In the months and years that followed Lisa's suicide attempt, she has taught us what the road to recovery looks like. She has experienced many things the system has to offer, including hospitalization in a mental health unit, adult day programming, emergency department crisis, mental health counseling, and doctor visits. Besides the help from the system, she continues to do everything she can herself to stay well. She takes her medications, keeps her appointments, gets enough sleep, eats well, exercises, and is mindful.

I am happy to report that in the past 8 years, she has returned to school, graduated, and now works permanently. Make no mistake, the road to recovery still has good days and bad days, but she has figured out a rhythm that works for her. We will be forever grateful.

This is the book I didn't want to write. Actually, I didn't want to write any book. I'm middle aged. Retirement is in view. We are empty nesters, all four children launched. Lisa is doing well. I have nothing left to prove to myself or anyone else. Quite a liberating time, indeed. But something kept gnawing inside me. Every day of my life since April 23, 2011, I frantically searched for answers. How does this happen? What can we do so it doesn't happen again to Lisa or anyone else? What about the ones that weren't so lucky? What about the loved ones who were left behind?

I have researched and read and probed on a daily basis. Even as a nurse who has witnessed many of life's complexities, I was dumbfounded. The more I dug in, the more I was perplexed. On the topic of suicide, there is a surprisingly large volume of research and many articulate scholars. There are many caring mental health professionals. Treatments are developing all the time with increasing success rates. There are suicide attempt survivors who have taught us so much. But why, why does this keep happening? What can we do to stop it? Then it hit me like a ton of bricks, the most painful truth I have ever faced in my life; we can't do it alone, everyone has to help. This book is my attempt to help.

2··WHAT?

Statistics

Suicide is a major cause of premature and preventable death worldwide. Every 40 seconds, somewhere in the world, someone ends their own life. Young people are the most affected. Suicide is now the second leading cause of death for those between the ages of 15 and 29.

Forty-five percent of all suicides are between the ages of 40 and 59. For every person who has completed suicide, there are 19 others that attempted. The suicide completion rate for males is three times higher than that of females, although females attempt suicide four times more than males. While the link between suicide and mental illness is well established, this percentage can fluctuate considerably depending on the country and the year (50-90%). Not everyone with a mental illness diagnosis has suicidal thoughts or attempts suicide. Suicide is rarely caused by any single factor. Other issues often contribute to suicide such as those related to relationships, substance use, physical health, jobs, money, or legal and housing issues.

Suicide affects certain segments of the population disproportionately, making some groups high risk. These include those with a mental illness diagnosis, minorities of race/ethnicity, previous suicide attempts, people bereaved by suicide, military personnel diagnosed with PTSD, sexual orientations of LGBTQ, and individuals who are incarcerated. No single determinant including mental illness is enough on its own to cause suicide, but rather it is the interaction of many factors; personal, social, psychological, cultural, biological, and environmental.

Some of the suicide warning signs that mean someone may be at risk include:

- Talking about wanting to die, or being preoccupied with death
- Talking about feelings of hopelessness or having no reason to live
- Talking about feeling trapped or in unbearable pain
- Talking about being a burden to others
- Increasing the use of alcohol or drugs
- Behaving recklessly, such as driving dangerously
- Seeking out lethal means
- Self-loathing, self-hatred
- Withdrawing or feeling isolated
- Displaying extreme moods
- Getting affairs in order

Suicide Myths

There are many myths that exist around suicide that stop people from getting help and stop others from helping. It's important to debunk the myths.

Myth: Talking about suicide will lead to or encourage suicide.

Fact: There isn't any research that indicates talking to people about suicide, in a caring respectful way, increases the risk of suicide incidents. In fact, research shows that talking about suicide reduces stigma, making it easier for individuals to seek help.

Myth: Most suicides happen without warning.

Fact: Warning signs – verbal or behavioral- precede most suicides. Many individuals who have suicidal thoughts do show outward signs.

Myth: People who die by suicide are selfish and take the easy way out.

Fact: Typically, people do not die by suicide because they do not want to live – people die by

suicide because their pain and suffering becomes overwhelming.

Myth: Someone who is suicidal is determined to die and there isn't anything that can be done to change their mind.

Fact: On the contrary, suicidal people are often ambivalent about living or dying.

Angus

My background is in nursing and I have spent my career doing home visits in the community. A very wise nursing professor once instilled in me that when you visit someone in their home don't ever forget you are a guest. They are King and this is their kingdom. You can be invited in or dismissed at any point. I never forget it.

One Friday, my last visit of the day was an elderly gentleman named Angus. He was referred from the local hospital after an admission for cardiac complications. He lived two miles down an unpaved road in an isolated area with no neighbors in view. I had been to Angus' home once before, two years earlier, but struck out when he didn't accept any help. I was dismissed from his kingdom like the court jester whose juggling act failed to impress. I was hoping for a better result today. I remembered Angus had a very quiet existence with limited social interaction. I remembered the last time he made me move my car when I pulled in because that's where the birds came to be fed. I wouldn't repeat that mistake.

Angus had lived alone in the old family home ever since his parents passed away many years before. When I knocked on the door, I heard a dog barking. It was then I remembered he had a dog. When Angus came to the door, I reminded him of our pet policy. The dog would need to be put in another room or leashed. Angus complied, leashed Sparky, and tied the leash to the leg of the table. Sparky, as described by Angus, was the smartest dog that ever lived. I didn't have to dig deep with my assessment skills to realize Sparky wasn't happy with me, an intruder in his home, nor in having his freedom infringed. Sparky eyeballed me like a protective father eyeballs his teenaged daughter's new boyfriend, reminding me, "I'm watching you."

As I made my way through my assessment, I realized Angus' recent setback was limiting his abilities to function in his usual life. I was hoping he would agree to some support in his home. When I asked him how his mood was, it led to a discussion on suicide, and had he ever thought about it. First, he said no, but then he nodded yes. He clarified, "sometimes I want for it all to end and sometimes I don't. Today I don't."

When I asked him what his plan was, he talked about the hunting rifle in his bedroom. How one -night last week he sat in the kitchen, holding the loaded gun." I would have done it, but who would look after Sparky?" he said.

We talked about access, and what can be done to get the gun out of the house, even for a short time. "I don't have anyone I can give it to, my family is all gone. I don't want to explain this to my neighbor. Did you want it?"

There were only two seconds between his question and my answer, but 20 separate thoughts went through my head. "I don't want this man to die and if the gun stays here he might; I might lose my job if I take it; what am I going to physically do with this gun; I have two small children I can't take it home; what if the police stop me on the way home how would I explain the gun in my car." Then I answered, "I'd love to have the gun."

He walked to his bedroom, a door off the kitchen and came out with his rifle. He was carrying it like a proud new mother carries her baby. He gave me a detailed explanation of how to use it when I go hunting, the perfect distance to stand, how to load it, and how to carry it safely.

He agreed I could call his family doctor and I did. He wouldn't agree to leave his home to see someone. The doctor would make a home visit and we agreed if the gun was gone, the risk was mitigated. I took the gun to the police station and told them my story. They arranged for the gun to be stored. Angus didn't want the gun back. I didn't lose my job. On my next visit, Sparky got a hero's breakfast.

What is Mental Health?

We can't begin a discussion on suicide without talking about mental health, declining mental health, and mental illness.

Good mental health could be described as functioning in our day to day lives without excess difficulty. When challenges arise, which they do in everyone's life, we work our way through them.

Declining mental health is when we are not able to work our way through our challenges as we did before. Mental illness causes significant changes to thinking, mood, and behavior for a period of time. Mental illness is a medical diagnosis, like diabetes and arthritis. I am not going to elaborate on any specific mental illness diagnosis. A diagnosis is given by a doctor and I am not a doctor (the degree on my wall confirms this).

A mental illness diagnosis comes from a book called the DSM (Diagnosis and Statistical Manual). The book has more than 300 diagnoses, weighs over three pounds, and is the work of hundreds of international experts. It is the lifeline of psychiatrists. There is a reason doctors go to university for so long. Some diagnoses that we might be personally familiar with or hear in the media are depression, anxiety, PTSD, bipolar, and substance abuse. The causes of mental illnesses can be multifactorial; our genetic predisposition, our environment, our biochemical makeup, our psychological functioning, and social factors.

What we do know about declining mental health is that regardless of diagnosis, it can present similarly, with changes to our mood, physical body, thoughts, and behavior. All these changes can contribute to a functional decline. That is how we function in day to day life. It might show up as being more irritable with our families. It might show up as missing deadlines at work. It might show up as having no energy to get out of bed in the morning. It might show up as having no appetite. It might show up as nagging back pain. It might show up with more negative thoughts.

The key to spotting mental health decline is being aware. It is recognizing that this is a change from your usual self. Maybe you were never a morning person, so not wanting to get out of bed in the morning is not a change. But if this is not your usual self, then take note of the change.

The statistics tell us that not everyone who attempts or completes suicide has a formal mental illness diagnosis. One of the biggest challenges and tragedy with the statistics is that many of the people that we need to ask are no longer with us. Did some of those individuals have a mental illness that wasn't diagnosed? What exactly was going on in their heads? Some of the best education we have is the information that we have obtained from the suicide attempt survivors, like Lisa. We know that for every twenty suicides attempted, only one is completed. A recurring story is there was some decline in the individual's mental health preceding the attempt, whether they had a formal mental illness diagnosis or not. This is why we will focus on mental health and the changes that can happen.

One of the best ways that I have discovered to explain mental health and mental health decline is on a continuum. When I say discovered I don't mean discovered in the same vein that Alexander Fleming discovered penicillin or Alexander Graham Bell discovered the telephone. There was no "Mr. Watson, come here, I want to see you," transmitted over copper wires. My discovery was more about sifting through existing work that had already been done by experts, finding ideas that I can understand, and passing these ideas on to anyone that will listen. No reinventing the wheel here.

Continuums are often used to help people understand complex topics with changes that happen insidiously. The changes vary by such tiny differences that over time it becomes difficult to follow when one is becoming the other. We often refer to health in general on a continuum. There is a fluid mechanics continuum in physics. There's no question mental health is every bit as complicated as any of the concepts in physics.

Many countries and academics have devised similar concepts when explaining mental health. The mental health continuum that I am using to explain mental health and mental illness is one that is used by the United States Marine Corp and Navy, The Canadian Mental Health Commission, and the Canadian Department of National Defense. No shortage of brains there. It was developed and revised to help mental health resiliency in the face of stressful situations like combat, stressful workplaces, and difficult situations in our lives. It uses a spectrum of mental health, where on one end you have good mental health and the other end you have poor mental health. In between the two ends you have varying degrees of changes. As with most continuums, the two ends are complete opposites.

good mental health	declining	poor mental health

One example that helps me understand the concept of a continuum is water and ice. On one end of the continuum, we have water, a free-flowing clear liquid. On the opposite end is ice, a hard solid. These are two very different states. Along the way, when one is moving closer to the other there are incremental changes; molecules slowing down, temperatures dropping, crystals forming, and less bumping and jostling. Sometimes these small changes are noticeable if you're paying attention, sometimes they're not. Also like our mental health, these states can move in both directions. Water can start to form ice, but at any point along the way, maybe with an increase in temperature or increased movement, it can go back to being free-flowing water. That's like our mental health, at any point along the way, with awareness, self-care and/or treatment, it can move back in the direction of good mental health.

A personal example of a continuum is our bank accounts. On one end of the continuum is our bank account on payday and the other end of the continuum is our bank account one day before the next payday. They are two opposites with lots of action along the way. There are expected bills such as mortgage, house utilities, phone and internet, car payment, gas, and groceries. There are some unexpected bills; tire repair from a blow-out, increase in insurance, the deck handrail that needed replacing. Then there are those expenses that feel like a surprise when we check our bank accounts that must have happened when we weren't paying attention. Was I at Starbucks nine times? That can't be right. Maybe the bank made a mistake? How many trips did I make to the grocery store? Seven feels like a lot. What did I even buy on Amazon? I'm sure that's a mistake. Then you remember the phone charger with the longer cord that arrived on Tuesday. Not an error at all. Then payday comes again, our bank account gets replenished and we move back on the continuum to a more positive economic outlook. So our bank account can be just like our mental health, sometimes the changes can be subtle, we might not even be aware that we are heading down on the continuum. Also like our bank accounts, we can change the direction of our mental health and move back to good mental health at any point along the way.

The Mental Health Continuum Model uses colors to group these changes that can occur along the line. Colors are used purposely to take away the stigma associated with labeling and specific diagnosis. It's so much easier to talk about sensitive topics when using a less emotionally charged label like a color. The colors are check in points that can help us figure out where we are. If we notice one color is changing to another color it can help us be aware of what's going on. Just like the bank account, if there was a check-in point early, maybe after 3 trips to Starbucks, it would have helped with awareness before the 9 trips were made.

There are four different colors in the continuum; green, yellow, orange, and red. Green is at one end of the continuum and red is at the opposite end. Green is described as healthy, adaptive, and coping. Yellow is next in line on the continuum and is described as reacting, self-limiting distress. Orange is the third grouping on the continuum, and it is described as injured, with more severe functional impairment. Red is on the opposite end and it is described as severe and persistent functional impairment, possibly a diagnosable mental illness that isn't being treated.

Green	Yellow	Orange	Red
healthy	reacting	injured	ill

Remember, like water and ice, your mental health functioning can decline and be heading to yellow or orange but can be reversed. Also, many people who have been in red with an untreated diagnosable mental illness, with awareness and treatment can recover and move back towards green. So, what might we notice in ourselves or others on the continuum when there is declining mental health?

Changes in Mood

Green	Yellow	Orange	Red
Your normal mood	Irritable	Angry	Easily enraged
Confident	Impatient	Anxious	Excessive anxiety
Calm	Nervous and sad	Pervasive sadness	Depressed and numb

Changes in Behavior and Performance

Green	Yellow	Orange	Red
Physically and socially active	Decreased activity and socialization	Avoidance and tardiness	Withdrawal and absenteeism
Performs duties/tasks well	Procrastination	Decreased performance	Can't perform
No impact due to alcohol and substance abuse	Some impact due to alcohol and substance abuse	Increased impact of alcohol and substance abuse	Significant impact of alcohol and substance abuse

Physical Changes

Green	Yellow	Orange	Red
Normal sleep	Trouble sleeping	Restless sleep	Can't fall or stay asleep
Good appetite	Changes in eating	Loss of appetite	No appetite
Feels energetic	Some lack of energy	Some fatigue	Constant fatigue
Maintains stable weight	Some weight gain or loss	Fluctuations or changes in weight	Extreme weight change

Changes in Thoughts

Green	Yellow	Orange	Red
Good sense of humor	Displaced sarcasm	Negative attitude	Suicidal thoughts with intent
Takes things in stride	Intrusive thoughts	Recurrent intrusive thoughts and images	Inability to concentrate
Ability to concentrate and focus on tasks	Easily distracted	Constantly distracted	Memory decline

Everyone looks a bit different on the mental health continuum. It's not exact; it's a guide. The signs and symptoms do not necessarily change together or in a precise pattern. It's approximate. It helps us be more aware. You might just have one symptom in a color, or you might have them all. One person may have sleep disturbances as their biggest symptom, and another may have changes in energy. Your appetite can be in yellow and your sleep in orange. Thoughts are the same. Your thoughts can become more negative on the continuum. It can be more difficult to concentrate, and your memory may get worse. You might have thoughts of suicide.

The key is to be aware of what's happening in our body and in our thoughts. At any point along the continuum we can make our way back to good mental health. We may need some help to do that.

Michael

I've had the good fortune of attending a yearly conference called "Living with Mental Illness and Addiction." It is an annual one-day event with over 500 people in attendance. The participants are a mix of health professionals working in mental health, professionals who don't specifically work in mental health, and the majority of the crowd is made up of individuals in the community with a mental illness diagnosis. The event is financially supported so there isn't any cost to participants. Lisa and I both look forward to attending yearly. It's a safe space for those that want to learn and share about mental health in any way.

There is always a keynote speaker at the conference who is a celebrity of sorts. There have been musicians, actors, actresses, military commanders, radio announcers, politicians, T.V newscasters, athletes, poets, and comedians. Their speeches are personal. They give us a glimpse into their celebrity world as we know it as outsiders. Then they give a glimpse into their world of living with a mental illness. This resonates deeply with the crowd. The crowd imagines that their life is so different from theirs and yet one part is so similar. There is comfort in that.

The keynote address is usually 45 minutes long and there is always a question period for 30 minutes after the speaker finishes. This is a time where individuals in the crowd are free to come to a microphone and ask questions. A bit like Reddit's AMA (ask me anything) without the safety net of the computer screen. Early in my career, I remember taking a course on presenting to the public. The seasoned instructor talked at length about how to handle questions from your audience, especially when your forum is open to the public. Some questions will completely rattle you, he said, you're not even sure what the person is asking or if it's even related in any way to what you're talking about. He called it "the speech in the back pocket." These are individuals in your audience who have their specific personal reason for being there and they've come to make it known to others. It happened to me twice before, in a prenatal class where a father was speaking about hidden arsenic in the water supply and at a caregiver support group where a caregiver was speaking about zoning bylaws. I was rattled. This conference brought out many speeches in the back pocket. Individuals feel this is a safe place and come to share something about their lives. Sometimes it's hard to figure if there's a question with their statement. I've seen experienced celebrities struggle with the open forum. It's not an easy task.

Four years ago, when I received the conference press release, I saw the keynote address was a man named

Michael Landsberg. I have to admit I didn't know who he was. I researched him online and saw he was the host of a sports show called "Off the Record" on TSN (The Sports Network), a national specialty cable network. He was the moderator of a half hour show featuring guests from sports and entertainment from different vantage points. Jamie yelled to me when he saw him come on TV that evening, "that's the guy who's speaking at the conference!"

I watched intently. He was opinionated and a bit in the face of the guests. He was called brash in his online intro. I was worried about how he would fit in at the conference. These people deserved the best. Jamie tried to explain this was his persona; part of his job to rile up the guests. It made it more entertaining. People aren't going to watch something if everyone agrees. Where's the fun in that? Maybe so, I thought, but I still wasn't convinced he was the right person for the conference.

From the time he walked on stage at the conference, he had the audience captivated. He told the story of his darkest time with mental illness and you could have heard a pin drop in the room.

"I was deep in the dark hole. It was Tuesday, November 24, 2008, at four in the morning and we were doing *Off the Record* at the Grey Cup. I had four sleepless nights. I was sitting on the edge of my bed thinking to myself, 'I know why people take their lives,' because I was in so much pain that I was aware that there was a finite amount of time that I could continue like that. That sense of hopelessness, that sense of loneliness. If I hadn't been through it before and knew that it would pass, it might have killed me. But it didn't."

"A year later I was interviewing former NHL player Stephane Richer, and I had read a small article where he had alluded to his mental health. Backstage before the interview, I asked how he would feel about me bringing up mental health in the interview. I said, 'I know that you struggled with depression in the 1990s. Would it be okay if I ask you how you're doing? and he said, 'I don't know, it's painful.' I told him that I had hard days too, and he was surprised. We went on the air and we talked for about a minute, when I asked how he was doing? He said: 'I'm doing a lot better.' And I said: 'I struggled too.' What followed was a candid conversation between two men about our mutual struggles."

"There was a flood of emails after the show. Many of them from men saying the same thing. This was the first time they've seen two men, talking openly about their mental health without shame, embarrassment, or seeming weak. They wanted to share their story with me. For some, it was the first time they're telling anyone, and it's with me in this email. This changed my life. That was the first time I shared in such a public way. It was then that I realized the power that we all have to use our platforms."

"So, two and a half years later, I had this moment, which I call my holy shit moment. Somebody who communicated with me after the Stephane Richer interview sent me another email. The email said: 'Hey, Michael you don't remember me, Tyson Wilson from North Battleford, Sask. Two and a half years ago, you and Stephane Richer talked about your struggles with depression. I messaged you and you messaged me back and we went back and forth five times. But what I didn't tell you was that my method was in my closet, I never told you what was going on. I never told you I was suicidal. I never told you the ping from you answering my email saved my life. I just told you that I didn't think that there was hope for me.' And you said, 'What do you have to lose if you go for help?'"

"'That changed my life because here I am, two and a half years later, able to celebrate my life.' Tyson added: 'Imagine, I had written a note to my daughter saying why I ended my life. How can this be?—a parent thinking my kid would be better off without me. I mean, no rational brain would think that.' He said: 'That's because a couple of guys shared.'"

After his 45 minutes of speaking, Landsberg opened questions from the floor. I have never seen a more engaged crowd, or any keynote speaker relate to the audience which such humility. He hit it out of the park. He handled the speeches in the back pockets like a pro. "Some days suck," he said, when they were done. They were heard.

Your Brain is a Liar

Psychologists and scientists tell us that our behaviors are a direct result of our thoughts. Our thoughts tell us that it is cold outside today, so we put on a jacket. Our thoughts tell us if we drive on the wrong side of the road, there will be an accident, so we drive on the right side. Our thoughts tell us if we put our hand on the stove burner when it is hot, we will get burned. So we don't put our hand on the burner. Our thoughts precede our actions. It's the same with suicide. A suicidal attempt is preceded by thoughts of suicide.

Thoughts are complicated. It is estimated that the average person has between 50,000 and 80,000 thoughts a day. I was thinking about how they even figured out that number. Some study participant in a research lab for 24 hours, marking a dash on a piece of paper every time they had a thought. Who would do that? Then I had a flash, 18-year old Shamus telling me he had just bought a new X-box. "Made two hundred dollars just sitting at a table-way better than working fast food." It's believable.

On the surface, it's hard to believe that we would have that many thoughts in a day. That is, until you try and learn to meditate. "Close your eyes and think about your breath," they say. Then you realize thinking about your breath is a nanosecond, and then it's interrupted with many separate thoughts; my arm is itchy, my foot isn't comfortable, what am I making for supper tonight, is this Thursday, what's on TV tonight, is today when the new Netflix special comes out, is there gas in the car?, did I lock my computer when I left work?, these pants aren't comfortable., the lavender is nice in the air freshener, etc. Some thoughts you don't even know where they came from, like the internet salesperson turning up at your door at suppertime - just there. Is she on breath in or breath out? This is just in the first 30 seconds. It quickly becomes clear that we are on autopilot most of the time. We are going about our days, doing our thing, thoughts coming and going, not even aware of most of them. So the statement "be aware of your thoughts" is far from easy.

Where do thoughts even come from? One article I found to explain thoughts suggested they were conditioned patterns. They are our ideas, opinions, and beliefs about ourselves and the world around us. They include our perspectives that we bring to any situation or experiences that color our point of view, which can be good, bad, or indifferent. The good can include all the positive things that have happened or are happening in our lives; playing games as a child, favorite teachers, times we were proud of ourselves, times our families were proud of us, a perfect cup of coffee this morning, and any moments of joy. Unfortunately, this pattern is also influenced by negative; schoolyard bullies, ingrained bad habits, mistakes from the past, unfounded beliefs, the car that cut you off in traffic this morning, memories of old traumas, and genetic susceptibilities. This all gets mixed in a big old hodgepodge to imprint our thoughts.

Twenty years ago, when Oprah recommended the book "The Power of Now" by author Eckhart Tolle, I immediately went out and bought the book. I admit I was a groupie of Oprah, watching her show daily and reading her recommended books like a faithful student. I laid in bed that night and started reading the book. I read the first three pages and I closed it. The message was "we are not our thoughts." That's the most ridiculous thing I ever read, I thought to myself. Plus, who's doing all the thinking if it's not me? Who's thinking they just wasted twenty dollars on this book? Pretty sure that's me. Oprah had disappointed. The last time Oprah had disappointed me was when she had a fashionista guest on her show, discussing women's summer trends when they said, "women over thirty shouldn't wear capris." Oprah nodded in agreement. There might not be any coming back from this second disappointment.

Fast forward fifteen years when I am frantically researching everything I can on how thoughts and suicide are related. Guess what? Eckhart Tolle, one of the most popular spiritual gurus in the world was right all along. We are not our thoughts. I read the book. It's a bit profound, but I'm getting there. One of his quotes that helped me understand this concept was, "what a liberation to realize the voice in my head is not who I am. Who am I then? The one that sees that." Sorry Eckhart and Oprah, I was wrong.

Our thoughts have a negativity bias. That is where we are neurologically wired to look for negative experiences over positive experiences. There is an evolutionary reason for this. Millions of years ago, it was a survival mechanism of our hunter-gatherer ancestors. It taught our ancestors to look favorably for danger/negative experience so they could anticipate a threat and their "flight or fight mechanism" would kick in, guaranteeing they would survive.

In fight or flight mechanisms, our energies get redirected so we can get away fast and our thoughts are completed focused on that escape, like wearing horse blinders. The hunter-gatherers that said, "aw, look, isn't that nice? So colorful, so pretty!" got eaten by a tiger. They weren't our relatives. They didn't survive to pass on their genes.

Our relatives were the negative Nellys, on guard for threats. "Did you hear that? I think I hear something in the brush, let's get out of here." They survived. That's the good part. The bad part is, the negativity bias is still very much in our brains. Even though the threats are less frequent in this modern world, our brains are in the state of high alert looking for danger. Ready to go. It makes seeing things in a negative light a whole lot easier than seeing things in a positive light. This negative narrative gets added to everyday events, which we accept as true. Blame the glass being half empty on your relatives.

Negative thoughts can lead to more negative thoughts. These inaccurate thoughts convince us that things sound logical when they're not. It's like the funhouse mirror at the carnival making something appear different than it is. We believe these thoughts to be true even when they aren't. These false and irrational thoughts get reinforced over time. These inaccurate thoughts have a fancy name - cognitive distortions. You've just met your liar.

Everyone has cognitive distortions. The individual difference is the degree to which we have them, and whether we consistently challenge them to test their validity. For example, every human has the thought that they are going to trip when going up on stage to receive a graduation diploma. For some, the thought is fleeting and passes when they remind themselves of the other times they've been on stage and didn't trip, and how infrequently tripping ever happens to them. For others, the tripping thought can be persistent, repeating the scenario over and over in their head until they become completely convinced it is going to happen. They believe the thought to be true and decide not to attend the graduation ceremony based on their belief.

These cognitive distortions have been grouped and named by clinicians to make them easier to spot. Some of the names include jumping to conclusions, all or nothing thinking, fortune telling, over-generalizing, catastrophizing, should statements, and personalization, to name a few.

Jumping to conclusions manifests as the inaccurate belief that we know exactly what another person is thinking. Someone walks by you at work and doesn't say hi after you said good morning. You jump to the conclusion that they hate you and you start reviewing scenarios in your head of why this is true. Did I leave the photocopier paper drawer empty? Building evidence, they were unusually quiet yesterday when I walked in the coffee room. The suggestion is that once we become aware of the distortion, we can challenge it. What is the evidence? Are there other possible interpretations? Maybe they didn't hear me it's quite loud in the hallways. Maybe they were preoccupied and rushing off to a meeting. With the challenge, we can see our thoughts aren't always true.

All or nothing thinking manifests as seeing things as black or white, unable to see shades of gray. You see things as extremes. Something is either fantastic or horrible. People are either good or bad. You write a challenging exam and when you leave, you tell everyone you failed it. If you didn't make 100, the only other option is failing. If you challenge this thinking, you could see there are many other possibilities between 50 and 100.

Catastrophizing or minimizing is the distortion where you either exaggerate the importance of an insignificant event or lessen the importance of a positive event. You back your car into the garbage container in your driveway. There isn't any damage to your car except for a scrape that can be buffed out. You continue to go over the scene many times in your head. How could I be so stupid? Why didn't I double check there wasn't anything there? I'm a terrible driver? I shouldn't even drive anymore, because I might cause a serious accident. What are the possible interpretations when you challenge the thought? I can still drive the car and you can't even notice the scrape. The garbage container was hidden by the tree branch. When we minimize, we take a positive thought like a promotion at work and minimize it. They probably had to give it me, nobody else must have wanted it. No thought that you were the best candidate because you are an exceptional employee.

Fortune telling is the distortion that manifests as the tendency to jump to conclusions or a negative prediction based on little or no evidence. It's like a crystal ball that only foretells a negative outcome. You take the prediction as a fact. You know the future with certainty and it's not good. Some research suggests that this distortion is uniquely associated with suicide attempt status. With research, we are always cautious when saying one thing proves something else until a large volume of work is done. In the meantime, if this distortion turns up in ourselves or we notice it in someone else, it is a red flag. It would be a prime suspect in any investigation. It's a red flag when someone always refers to the future with dread. They may use words such as never; I will never feel better, I can never do it right, work will never get any better. When I read over the things that Lisa told us about her thoughts when she felt better, I can see the fortune teller; my family and friends would be better off without me, there isn't any help that will make a difference, no one can make a difference. We need to be aware of this distortion and challenge it. Where is the evidence? What are the other possible outcomes? It can get better. Others have felt the same way and now they say it gets better. There is hope.

The difference in the outcome of the cognitive distortions is a result of challenging of the negative thoughts. Some people can challenge them easier than others. In declining mental health, it becomes more difficult to challenge these distortions (lies). The lies become more believable when they're not true. One of the prime treatments for declining mental health is cognitive behavior therapy (CBT). This is a treatment that focuses on being aware of these thoughts and teaches people how to challenge and test their validity. It teaches you skills to tackle negative thoughts like a skilled lawyer would disprove allegations against his client. Where's your proof? This isn't true and I'll show you why not! In CBT when we challenge our negative thoughts, we are actually making new pathways in our brain. We are essentially rewiring our own brain.

Chen

After university, when the recession was in full surge, Jamie and I moved to an isolated small mining town north the 56th parallel. We were only too happy to live where we both could have full-time jobs. The town was literally the "end of the road" where the highway came to an abrupt end. Winters were cold. I had lucked my way into working as a Public Health Nurse. Chen and Nick were a mid-twenties couple who had attended my prenatal class, every Wednesday evening for eight weeks. Chen was a teacher. Nick was an information systems engineer. We had a similar trajectory. Newlyweds making our way in the world, far from our families. Chen and Nick were so excited to be expecting a baby, asking every question possible to prepare them for the next milestone in their lives.

After the baby was born, I got to make a home visit. One of the special perks of being a public health nurse. Baby Aurora Jane was a beautiful 7lb 6-ounce bundle. Things seemed to be going well. The baby was gaining weight and now at 95th percentile, no issues with breastfeeding, said the chart notes.

The next time I saw them was when Chen brought Aurora to our clinic to get her two-month immunization. There was lots of chatter about Aurora's developmental milestones; smiling more and holding her head steadier. She had stopped breastfeeding; it was getting too hard. Aurora was still up in the night. When I asked, "How's mom doing?" It was a roundabout conversation that eventually got to "Not very good. I had wanted this baby so badly and now I feel like a failure. I'm a terrible mother. Aurora hates me. She would be better off without me. I'm crying all the time. I'm so tired. I'm lying on the couch, still in my pajamas when Nick gets home from work. This was a mistake. I keep having these fearful thoughts in my head about hurting myself. I just want this horrible pain to stop. I'm scared. I need my mom. I don't even know how I would explain this to Nick." We talked about how sometimes this happens. She was a great mother, just needed some help. I called her doctor and he would see her right away. We called Nick together and he came to pick them up.

A year later I ran into Chen and Aurora at the grocery checkout. Aurora was the picture of health, not only walking, but now running. As they scurried out the door Chen turned back and said, "Hey, thanks for everything. You were right, I am a good mother."

Suicidal Thoughts

Suicidal thoughts have their own name, Suicidal Ideation, SI, in abbreviated form. Suicidal Ideation can be fleeting and passive at one end, such as a four-second mental image of your funeral after fighting with a loved one (they'll be sorry they were mean). On the other end, which requires professional assessment, are suicidal thoughts with a detailed plan. The more details, the more of an emergency. In between the two ends, as things get worse, there is a progression involving more details.

The part that's hard to get our heads around is when a suicide attempt or completion appears to come out of the blue. No one saw it coming. What you have to remember is that our thoughts are in our heads. There might be things happening to the individual that isn't apparent to those around them. The person themselves might not even have full awareness. They might, and they might not, have a mental illness diagnosis. They might have some of the risk factors. They might already be in orange or red on the continuum. They might be sleeping poorly, eating poorly, have predominantly negative thoughts in their head. They might have suicidal thoughts in some way for some time, but don't have any specific plan. They might be using alcohol or drugs to excess in order to numb their pain. All these things are accumulating. Then one thing happens; divorce papers arrive, they lose a job, a relationship breakup, or in Lisa's situation, a failed academic year. To most, these situations might seem like one of life's disappointments, unfortunate, but manageable. To the already distressed person, it's the tipping point, the straw that breaks the camel's back. It's the cumulative effect of many different things.

It is thought that many suicide attempts occur with little planning during a short-term crisis. A suicidal crisis is a temporary state that occurs in response to overwhelming stress, which is associated with unbearable emotional pain. The pain is perceived to be so severe and all-encompassing that no other solution can be thought of. The suicide attempt can be impulsive in the crisis moment during heightened duress (when the straw breaks the camel's back).

Our bodies are physically responding during this hyperarousal using the "fight or flight mechanism" that activates our sympathetic nervous system. This was passed on from our hunter-gatherer ancestors. When our ancestors perceived an attack or threat to their survival, they responded by either fleeing or fighting back. Both of these activities involve increased strength, muscle tension, and energy. By redirecting our hormones and neurotransmitters, our heart, lungs, and muscles are ramped up. The circuits were designed to get the body moving fast. The downside is what is thought to be our nonessential systems are shut down to divert the energy to the emergency functions. Unfortunately, one of the systems that shuts down is the rational, logical thinking from our brains. It is called cognitive constriction. This is why impulsive acts can happen during heightened duress as our logical thinking is shutting down. Problem-solving is difficult.

Dr Christine Moutier, chief medical officer of the American Foundation of Suicide Prevention explains what is actually happening in the brain in a suicidal crisis. "It is called cognitive constriction and the actual physiological functioning of the brain changes. There is a narrowing of coping options that stems from changes in the brains ability to come up with three or four ideas to problem solve, like it usually would. Cognitive constriction is often described as a feeling of tunnel vision, as if you were seeing through a straw, or wearing blinders. This is why we hear suicide attempt survivors say phrases like "I thought it was my only way out." This also dispels the myth that people who die by suicide are weak or selfish; in that state, they can't see beyond their circumstances. The mental distortion isn't permanent, but people can't see that in the moment. The transient nature of the physical change is why if people can live through it, they regain their usual coping functions and survive long beyond that moment."

In one study of suicide attempt survivors, the researchers asked," how much time passed between the time you decided to complete suicide and when you attempted?" Twenty-four percent were under five minutes, and 48% were under 19 minutes, suggesting a short, intense period of duress. Statistics also indicate the only 15% of individuals who complete suicide leave a suicide note, suggesting for the majority the action happened quickly. Suicide-attempt survivors often report that even when the suicide attempt was planned and not impulsive, they are often indecisive about the action. There is often a struggle with ambivalence. Self-preservation is one of our basic instincts that have ensured the survival of our species. Kevin Hines is a suicide attempt survivor who recounts his experience of jumping off the Golden Gate Bridge and surviving. Over 2000 people have used the Golden Gate Bridge as a suicidal means and the survival rate is less than 3%. It is a lethal means. Kevin relays he had a very specific plan. He knew where he was going that day. He took a city bus to the bridge, but he was still indecisive." I actually had a pact with myself, if one person says, are you OK, is something wrong, or can I help you? I was going to tell them everything and beg them to help me. The millisecond my legs cleared the bridge, the millisecond of true freefall, I had instant regret for my action. My first thought was what in the hell did I just do, I don't want to die."

Another Golden Gate Bridge suicide attempt survivor Ken Baldwin had a similar insight. "I just vaulted over, and I realized, at that moment, this is the stupidest thing I could have done. I immediately thought of my wife and my daughter."

There is a myth that if a person is suicidal, they are determined to die and there isn't anything that can be done by themselves or others to change the outcome. This is a myth and not true. We know that these thoughts happen. We know that the intensity of the thoughts will pass. We know that it's a basic instinct to stay alive. What can we do with this information to help ourselves and each other?

Immediate Actions

Get help right away.

Please tell someone if these thoughts give you ideas or plans to do something permanent. Don't be embarrassed and don't be afraid. There is help if you reach out. You do not have to face this alone. Please tell someone; your mom, your friend, your spouse, your teacher, your doctor, your therapist, or call a suicide crisis line. They will understand. There are numbers in the back of this book. Telling someone what's going on is the best way to get help.

Separate yourself from the means in the moment.

If you get caught in a moment of heightened duress, try to separate yourself from the suicidal means. Remember the time period can be very short from heightened duress to action. If you have pills in your hands and have the thought to swallow the whole bottle, flush the pills quickly down the toilet. If you are in a triggering location, such as a house where you know there's a gun, leave the home. The idea is to "buy time." It is known that the intensity of the thought will pass fairly quickly. The more you can do to let time pass, the better the chance of surviving.

Take deep breaths.

If you feel a crisis escalating, try to breathe deeply after you've called for help and separated yourself from the means. Deep breathing activates our parasympathetic nervous systems and tricks our body into believing that we are relaxed. It can deactivate the fight or flight mechanism and calm our bodies down. It releases the cognitive constriction and allows our brains to think logically again.

Preventative Measures

Be aware.

Two simple words that can be very hard to do. Remember the mental health continuum from earlier showing how our mood, behavior, physical health, alcohol and drug use, sleep, and thoughts can decline. With suicidal attempts, it is suggested that the individual's mental health had been declining. There is often a large number of things happening that progress on the continuum. Therefore, the earlier you notice a decline or change, the earlier you should go for help. Maybe you notice you're yellow in the continuum, some small changes, but things are not getting any better. This might be the time to talk to a professional like your family doctor. They might suggest interventions like exercise, therapy, relaxation interventions, adapted sleep hygiene, meditation, or medications, if necessary.

Research suggests the earlier we treat a decline, the easier it is to treat. Most times, with treatment we can halt a progression and send it back in a positive direction with interventions. Continue to check in with yourself to see if you notice things changing. Remember, these changes may or may not be noticeable to other people. However, if someone familiar to you mentions that they have noticed a change in your regular function, take notice. Sometimes, we might be on autopilot and not notice changes that are happening in ourselves. Remember the nine trips to Starbucks. Sometimes on the continuum, our level of self-awareness also declines. So if someone brings something to your attention - take note.

Make a safety plan.

If you recognize that your mental health is declining and you've had even occasional thoughts of suicide, then the idea is to write out some simple notes to yourself that you can refer to in an emergency. Since we know that it can be harder to problem solve and think clearly in a crisis, keep the notes concise and in a place where you can find them in a hurry. Store them in the notes section of your phone, a written note in your wallet or by your bed. If you share this information with your therapist or psychiatrist, they can help you write the note, but you can also do it yourself. In the note, write the name of three people that you trust and their phone numbers that you could call in a crisis. Write the numbers for your doctor and therapist. Write the number for a suicide crisis line for your local area. You can also program these numbers into your cell phone. There are also some apps that exist that you can download and keep on your phone that can help with a safety plan; MY3, Stay Alive, Operation Reach Out, etc. Having a safety plan does not make you weak, it makes your smart. More than likely, you will never have to use it, but if you do, it's there.

Make the environment safe.

We need to spend some time thinking about how to limit access to suicidal means in our homes. Restricting access to the means for suicide is a key component of suicide prevention efforts. This provides an opportunity for these individuals to reflect on what they are about to do and, hopefully, for the crisis to pass.

This is one example of how access to means was effective in preventing suicides in Britain.

For generations, the people of Britain heated their homes and fueled their stoves with coal gas. This coal-derived gas could also be deadly as it released very high levels of carbon monoxide. An open valve or a closed space could induce asphyxiation in a matter of minutes. This extreme toxicity also made it a common method of suicide. "Sticking one's head in the oven" became so common in Britain that by the late 1950s, it accounted for almost half the nation's means of suicide. Over the next decade, the British Government phased out coal gas in favor of natural gas. During these same years, Britain's suicide rate dropped by a third and it has remained at this lower rate. It is thought that this indicated that people who asphyxiated themselves did so impulsively in a moment of despair. Removing the oven slowed down the process allowing time for second thoughts and time for the despair to pass.

Another example of how access to means affected the suicide rate is the use of pesticides. In many lower-income countries, suicide rates are related to the accessibility of pesticides used in farming. Pesticides are typically stored within easy reach at home. In Sri Lanka, where a national pesticide ban was put in place, suicide rates dropped considerably. This suggests that limiting access to a quick means has positive outcomes.

We know that when a lethal means is used, there is a higher rate of suicide completion. We need to safeguard our homes and identify any lethal means.

If we know that we have thought about using a specific means then we need to do some advance planning to ensure the means is not available, or that it is somewhere that it's going to take time to access. That's not being weak, that's being smart. For example, if you have thought about taking an overdose of medications, then you should limit the number of pills you have access to at any one time. Having a one- or two-day supply of medications available and the rest in a lock box could work. Maybe your pharmacy could dispense medications for a limited period. Also, we can limit the amount of over the counter medications we have in the home at any one time. Get a small bottle as opposed to buying super-sized anything.

We need to think about our access to a gun. A gun is a lethal means. It very rarely gives a second chance. It rarely buys you time for heightened duress to pass giving less opportunity to reconsider. Guns are why the male suicide completion rate is higher than female when females attempt four times as often. In the US in 2015, over 50% of the completed suicides were from guns. Parents own the majority of guns that were used in teenage suicides by firearms. What can we do about a gun in our home? If someone in your home has declining mental health (yellow, orange or red), you need to think about the gun. Maybe the gun should be removed, even for a period of time. If that isn't possible, we need to think about what actions we can take ahead of time to buy some time for the person in heightened duress. Could the gun be locked with the key held by one person? Could the gun and the ammunition be separated (different floors of the house, ammunition in the shed)? A veteran client who acknowledged suicidal thoughts at times, once told me that he keeps his gun in his house, but no ammunition on his property. He knows he would have to get in his car, drive across town to the hardware store in daytime hours to buy ammunition. Essentially buying some time.

I grew up in a rural area in a family of eight children. These were days before parenting books and online parenting advice blogs. My mom was a stay at home mother, and my dad worked in the coal mines. My older brother John had a hunting rifle that he bought at age 16. Every Friday evening my parents would go by themselves to the nearest town to go grocery shopping. The seventies version of date night; groceries and a hamburger, home by eight. One Friday I noticed my mom putting the bolt from the gun and the package of bullets in her purse before she left. I thought about this action over the years and wondered if she was overly concerned about one of us. Last month I asked my mom about it. This was the response of my very wise 87-year-old mother, "No particular concern, just no sense looking for trouble leaving a house full of teenagers and a usable gun." Maybe we all just need to think pragmatically about the gun.

Be careful self-medicating with alcohol or drugs.

It is not uncommon for someone with declining mental health to use alcohol or drugs to temporary feel better by "numbing the pain." Acute alcohol or drug intoxication is present in a large number of suicide attempts. Alcohol and some drugs can cause impaired judgement and impulsivity. They have a disinhibiting effect on our thinking. It impairs our natural instinct for self-preservation. Think about the type and the amount of alcohol and drugs we have access to in our homes. Should they be limited? Should they be locked? It might be prescription pain killers belonging to people in the home or at grandparents' homes. Try to limit access to means as best you can.

3··HOW?

Use Your Platform

While most of us are not going to walk the red carpet on our way to winning an Oscar (sorry for the shock), we all have our own unique platforms. This is where we interact with other people. Your platform may be your family and friends. It might be your workplace. It might be sports or social clubs you belong to. It might be your social media connections. It could be your once monthly group of stamp collectors or your weekly Zumba class. It might be an online gaming group. It doesn't matter what the group is. It's anywhere that people engage. Wherever your platform is, it has power. It can reach people. The ask is to use your platform to talk about mental health in a positive way whenever an opportunity arises.

While we are asking anyone with mental health concerns to "reach out", the flip side of that is "reaching in." Sometimes mental health decline takes away perspective, energy, and motivation. Their brain is telling them that no one cares, or no one can help. Reaching out can seem like the most difficult thing in the world. Reaching in is what we can do and doesn't have to be hard at all. It might be offering to pick up a quart of milk for your neighbor who`s decline has stopped her from going to the grocery store. It might be asking someone, are you OK? Then truly listening to the answer. It may be staying in on Friday night, watching a movie with your friend, who hasn't followed through on plans to go out socially the last 6 times. There is no perfect script of what to do or what to say. Anything that you do from a genuine and caring part of you is never wrong.

We know that mental health stigma is one of the most debilitating challenges. Mental illness has negative stereotypes and they are ingrained. Over the years, media and movies have depicted mental illness in a negative light. Think of how mental illness was characterized in the movie, One Flew Over the Cuckoo's Nest and the movie, Psycho. Stigma is often the reason people don't ask for help. Stigma is often the reason people deny something is wrong, even to themselves. In the movie, Steel Magnolias, Shirley MacLaine plays a cranky character named Ouiser. When Ouiser is asked about her mood by her friend M'Lynn (Sally Field) she replies, "I've just been in a very bad mood for forty years." That's a long time to be in a bad mood.

It is suggested that less than half of people with a diagnosable mental illness actually go for help. We know that going for help makes a difference. While there can be other barriers to seeking help such as knowledge, access, and cost, the biggest barrier is without a doubt, stigma. Sometimes the words we use perpetuate stigma. Words such as; crazy, lunatic, nuts, wacky, insane, schizo, psycho, bonkers, nutcase, deranged, and loony exist in our everyday conversations. They're there. They're hurtful. We use them out of habit without even thinking of their connotations. Even when we are aware that we shouldn't use them, they can slip out. I'm surprised myself when expressions such as "what a crazy day, or that's a crazy amount of money" just slips out. Words are powerful. We need to be careful. We can do better. Just by watching our own words we can help with stigma.

Multiple research studies suggest that when an employee is off work due to mental health difficulties, the biggest obstacle to returning to work is the stigma in their workplace. Their biggest obstacle in returning to work was not their issues with fatigue, memory, concentration, pain, sleep, appetite, or negative thoughts. Their biggest obstacle was the judgment of their coworkers and managers when they returned (employers take note). We can do something about that. It doesn't have to be complicated. Your coworker returns after being off work for a month maybe just say "it's good to see you back", or "how's it going", or "just ask me if you need any help with the new (expense account, monthly stats, purchase order, phone system, etc.,) that started when you were off", or "we're going out to lunch on payday if you're around." I know you are thinking how I know if they have been off because of their mental health when they haven't told me. I don't want to intrude in their business. If you say, "it's good to see you back" no one is going to be offended and say, "how dare you, I was off with my gallbladder, you idiot." It still works. A kind gesture impacts everyone who observes it. Maybe it will even inspire others to be kind too. Small gestures make a big difference in helping fight stigma.

A byproduct of stigma is discrimination. Discrimination is negative actions toward people on the basis of their perceived group, like mental illness. Pam is the best candidate for the manager's job and has self-identified as having a mental illness. The stereotype exists that having a mental illness somehow makes you less capable. There is no truth to the stereotype. She is passed over for the job. That's discrimination. That's the action that happened as a result of stigma. Don't be a part of it. Even if you see the discrimination being parceled as something else, "We just don't think Pam's conceptual skills are the right fit and her score was lower in the interview." You all know that Pam's management and leadership skills greatly exceed all the other candidates and the interview questions were subjective. Discrimination would be hard to prove. Speak up if you see it happening. Use your power and challenge the thinking of others.

Remember earlier in the book, risk factors for suicide were noted. Suicide affects certain segments of the population disproportionately, making some groups higher risk. Reread the list. A large number of the groups in the list face discrimination, those with mental illness, minorities of race/ethnicity, sexual orientations of lesbian, gay, bisexual, transgendered, queer and incarcerated individuals. We need to do what we can in our platforms to prevent discrimination. Every small action helps.

Lots has been written about social media and mental health and some of it is negative. Social media is powerful, and its platform is far reaching. Be like Superman and use your power for good and not evil.

There can be educational material, positive encouragements, and support in communities on social media. People can feel less alone. Please promote the positive. There is also a negative side to social media. How many times have we seen posts on Facebook stating we're throwing away money helping addiction issues, or how people in prison are living the life of luxury? It's complicated. I can't explain it all. Likely, these are just good people who made a few more mistakes than the rest of us. You have no idea who is reading your post in cyber-world. When you see something negative or stereotypical please don't like, share, or retweet. Silence can help stigma. It can be a form of public condemnation. People get the idea when there aren't any likes. It's like Justin Timberlake sings, "Sometimes the greatest way to say something is to say nothing at all."

Promote kindness on your platform, always. There's even a payoff for being kind. No, there's not a new car sitting in your driveway from Oprah. It's better than that. Many research studies are now suggesting that being kind to others contributes to our own overall happiness, in a big way. It also significantly boosts our health and inadvertently makes us more successful. That's a good payoff. You're welcome.

A special thank you to the celebrities who have used their platforms in a positive way to promote mental health. This is huge. Sometimes I wonder if they even realize how powerful this is. Thank you to many musicians whose lyrics speak to those struggling and help people feel less alone. Thank you to the comedians who use self-deprecating humor to make a painful situation a little more bearable. Thank you to the actors and actresses that played roles in movies that depict mental illness in its realistic form. Lisa and others are comforted by your actions. Thank you to all the celebrities who have helped by sharing their own personal stories; Justin Bieber, Hailey Bieber, Alanis Morissette, Lady Gaga, Ellen DeGeneres, Demi Lovato, Selena Gomez, Catherine Zeta Jones, Adele, Brooke Shields, Ariana Grande, Ryan Reynolds, Kristen Bell, Anderson Cooper, Chrissy Teigen, Dan Harris, Halle Berry, Sarah Silverman, Pete Davidson, Beyoncé, Jessica Simpson, Prince Harry, Prince William, Miley Cyrus, Mariah Carey, Glenn Close, Winona Ryder, J.K. Rowling, and Gwyneth Paltrow. The list goes on.

Sharing is never easy, especially for someone in the public eye. There are risks. Sometimes the public is fickle, and haters do exist. But they did it anyways.

So thank you. In Ellen's Netflix special called "Relatable," she tells the story of "coming out" in Hollywood twenty years ago. She lost her sitcom as a result. Prior to her daytime talk show, she was told "no one's going to watch a lesbian during the day." She survived. She thrived. Yes, Ellen, you are more relatable then you will ever know. Thank you.

Lastly, the biggest ask is for everyone with lived experience. Whether you realize this or not, you have a superpower that others don't have. It's not that we don't need doctors, therapists, our family, friends, medications, exercise, meditation, cognitive behavior therapy, and many other helpful interventions. Yes, we need them all, too. What lived experience can give is hope to those struggling, and hope is a superpower. It sends the fortune teller packing (the one who was so certain of a negative future). When people struggling hear you talking about how you manage your hard days, and how some days suck, but other days are good, they're listening. When you relay how there was a time you wondered if it would get better and then it did, you give people hope. You give people courage and hope and belief in themselves that they are going to be OK, and that they can do this too. Thank you to the everyday people, who in their own way, share their story. Please continue. We are grateful.

Lisa

My name is Lisa MacDonald and I'm 28 years old. When I was growing up, I had a great childhood with a loving family and many friends. In my early teens, I remember starting not to like myself anymore and not feeling good enough. It was harder to concentrate at school. I was so tired. My legs and arms felt like they were made of lead. I constantly had an empty feeling in my stomach and sometimes I felt like someone was standing on my chest.

I started having thoughts that scared me and I tried to distract myself to make them go away. I didn't understand what was happening and that made me feel alone. I thought I was the only one who felt this amount of pain when nothing major was going on. I started to feel that no-one could understand or even care. I didn't know anyone who was like me.

I started to self-harm. My parents made me go to counseling, which I resisted for a while. I was fourteen. I didn't want some stranger knowing what I was thinking; I didn't even have words to explain it anyways. I took medication, and for a while, I did feel better.

When I was 19, I thought I was well enough to go away to college. Being away from my family and friends, plus living on my own and trying to do school, became too much. I started to slip. I denied to myself that I was sinking this far down again. Lots of days, I didn't get out of bed. I didn't shower. I didn't eat. I was failing school. I started to think about dying constantly. I researched methods. It consumed my thoughts. I didn't tell my family or therapist. I was living a lie. I had become a great actress. Pretending to be okay when all I wanted to do was disappear forever.

Things were snowballing and I felt like I had nowhere to turn. I could not see outside my illness and realize that I had friends and family I could turn to. I felt like I had no choice, that ending it all was the only way. I believed it wouldn't get better. I thought that my family, friends, boyfriend, and the whole world would be better off without me. I believed I was a huge burden. I thought to myself "if nothing will get better, then I'll have to live the rest of my life this way, and I can't do it."

I thought to myself that if I was dead my family wouldn't have to worry about my ups and downs. I didn't care about myself. I didn't think I was worthy of life. I didn't think I deserved to be happy. My thoughts of suicide became obsessive and unbearable. Thoughts just kept repeating in my head, over and over; you're ruined, you deserve to suffer, you're worthless, you're a failure, it's not going to get better. I just wanted the pain to stop. I was trapped in my own head. It started to comfort me knowing that soon it would be over, and the pain would finally stop.

One evening it all came to a head. I smoked some weed to calm myself. I went into the woods, and that's where I did it.

The next thing I remember is waking up on the ground and realizing it wasn't over. It was dark and cold. I could hardly breathe. I could see my phone in the distance reflecting the moon. I crawled to it and dialed 911. I cried to the operator on the line saying, I want to live, I want to be found, I'm sorry, please help me. The next thing I remember is seeing a flashlight beam and a dog leading police to me. I was taken to the hospital by ambulance and that's where my healing began.

After I was discharged from hospital, I went into a day program with other people living with mental illness. It was an amazing experience. I had never talked so openly about my illness before. I got to hear others speak freely about their lives. The details were different, but the challenges were the same. There was such comfort in realizing that others had suffered in similar ways. I couldn't believe that there were people who could relate to me. It didn't matter if they were a middle-aged professional man, a new mother, a grandmother, or a teenager. It didn't matter if they were rich or financially strapped. The feelings were the same.

For the first time since becoming ill, I no longer felt alone. There was such support. There was such hope. There was laughter. We all worked hard. There were caring professionals and new coping strategies. We were taught to challenge our negative thoughts, do deep breathing, exercise, eat healthy, meditate, manage our sleep, identify our emotions, pay attention to what our bodies are telling us, make time for healthy recreation, identify our triggers, and most important to ask for help.

That was eight years ago. Since then I have been doing so much better. It's not perfect, but I have an amazing life that I never could have envisioned eight years ago. I went back to school. I work full time. I provide peer support to those struggling. I take my medications, keep my medical appointments, and try to practice the coping strategies that I learned. I got a tattoo that says "this too shall pass" as a reminder that, although things might seem bad at the time, it will pass. As soon as symptoms appear, I keep my family, boyfriend, therapist, and doctor in the loop. I don't wait for things to get out of control before I take action.

I have learned so much in my recovery. I've learned this isn't my fault. I've learned there isn't one easy solution and feeling better takes patience. I've learned I need to love and take care of myself, and to pay attention to what my body is telling me. I've learned I need positive and stable relationships with the people I choose to spend time with. I've learned to express my emotions in a healthier way and be open about how I'm feeling. I've learned to ask for help. I've learned that just because things don't go as planned, it doesn't mean I'm a failure. I've learned that sharing my story helps others. Most of all I've learned my life is valuable and I no longer live in shame.

If you're reading this and you're struggling, I want you to know that it is never too late to get help. I want you to know your life is valuable. I want you to know that even when things seem completely hopeless it can get better. I want you to know that your mind can tell you things that aren't true. You are irreplaceable and your presence makes a difference in the world, whether you believe it or not. You CAN get through this. You are not alone.

Ideas Worth Stealing

USA

In 2001, the Henry Ford Health System in Detroit Michigan pioneered a formal program to reduce suicides to zero among their population. Their goal was to develop care pathways and modify the suicide risk. Primary care doctors started screening every patient that came to their office for depression, regardless of the purpose of the visit. Patients who came up positive in the screening were encouraged to try talk therapy or group counseling. Medication or hospitalization was considered if warranted. The administration staff were trained to make sure every patient who needed follow up got an appointment. Therapists involved patient's families and asked that guns or other means of suicide were removed from their homes. Patients wrote their own safety plan. Suicide rates dropped and remain 80% lower than before the program was started. In 2009, they registered zero suicides for the year.

Canada

In Sydney, Nova Scotia, an annual conference is organized titled "Living with Mental Illness and Addiction." This conference is organized by a partnership with the provincial health authority, individuals, and families with mental health and addiction issues and community organizations. The conference is open to professionals and those living with mental illness and addiction issues in the community. A concerted effort is made to reach and encourage participants from the community. It is free to attend, and coffee breaks and lunch are provided. It provides a full day of education and first- person experiences.

Australia

Jeffrey Forbes an Australian tradesperson was saddened when another fellow "tradie" died by suicide. Suicide rates in the tradie community were higher than all other occupations combined. He was determined to do something to help other tradespeople who he knew were suffering. They were expected to be strong, robust, macho, and silent in the face of adversity. He knew it wouldn't be easy to get them to take part in any formal education, but he needed them to attend. He worked with local communities. The end result was educational sessions held before 9am and after 5pm, providing convenient times that wouldn't reduce their income. Local and national mental health resources were provided. Local businesses provided donations of food. The sessions were provided in familiar locations to the tradies such as hardware stores and sheds. There have been over 150 sessions providing a comfortable place to open up and start a conversation on suicide.

Canada

Statistics tell us that many individuals that attempt suicide have contact with the healthcare system in the week or month preceding the attempt. The contact might not be related to an obvious mental health issue. It could be any number of nonspecific complaints such as; sleep difficulties, aches and pains, headaches or low energy. A health professional like a family doctor already has established a trusting relationship and they are often best positioned to identify those who may be at risk for suicide. Since mental health is not their specialty the Mental Health Commission of Canada, MDbriefcase and the Canadian Association for Suicide Prevention have developed on online accredited suicide prevention module for professional staff. This extra training helps physicians and nurses be more comfortable having these conversations with their patients. This helps identify those who need more follow up with a mental health professional. The free online training can be done in a few hours at their desk or home computer and are accredited for continuing professional development

USA

In the late 1960s, Dr. Jerome Motto, a psychiatrist in San Francisco, devised a research project aimed at suicidal patients who refused any treatment and didn't want any further contact with the health system. He argued that even the most despondent could still be reached. His subjects were divided into two groups. The contact group received a typewritten form letter, one or two sentences that were personally signed by the researcher. The letters expressed an interest in the subject without making any demands. They were sent monthly, and then quarterly for five years. They had notes such as: "it's been some time since you were here at the hospital, and we hope things are going well for you. If you wish to drop us a line, we would be glad to hear from you," or "this is a note to say we hope things are going well, as we remain interested in your well-being. Drop us a line anytime you like," or, "we realize that receiving a letter periodically expressing our interest in how things are going seems a bit routine, however, we continue to be interested in you and how you are doing."

There were no expressions that made demands like, "you need to call and make an appointment to resume therapy," or "your appointment is February 10th at 2:30," or "would you fill in this questionnaire and mail it back." There were just letters that showed genuine interest. Many letters were not answered.

Mott described his most pivotal response as one from a patient who had written a "kiss off" letter 18 months earlier. The letter was five typed pages long that started with "you are the most persistent son-of-a-bitch I've ever encountered, so you must really be sincere in your interest in me." Motto called this letter the perfect encapsulation of the study's aim. The bingo letter.

The research data showed that the contact group that received "caring letters" had half the number of further suicide attempts than the control group. He had demonstrated that people who had attempted suicide and wanted nothing to do with the mental health system could still be reached.

Conclusion

So that's it. This is what I've learned in the past eight years that helps me sleep at night. It's not easy. When our mental health declines, our thoughts lie to us and can tell us horrible things that aren't true. Suicidal thoughts exist and are more common than I ever imagined. They give us warning. It's like the check engine light coming on in our car to alert us that something needs immediate attention. Something is not right. You need to pull over and get help.

Stigma keeps people from getting help and treatment helps. It can get better and there is hope. There are things we can do ahead of time to prepare us for a crisis when our brains aren't thinking straight. In a crisis, get help, buy time, and breathe. We need you. There's work to be done. Be kind. Together we can send suicide packing. Lisa and I say thanks for helping.

Crisis Lines

CANADA

Canada Suicide Prevention Service: 1-833-456-4566 available 24/7

Kids Help Phone: 1-800-668-6868

Youth crisis text line: text TALK to 686868

Adult crisis text line: text 45645

Number for emergency: 911 anywhere in Canada

USA

National Suicide Prevention Lifeline: 1-800-273-8255 available 24/7

National Hope Helpline: 1-800-784-2433 available 24/7

Youth American Hotline: 1-877-968-8454

Veterans Crisis Line: 1-800-273-8255

Ulifeline for college and university students: 1-800-273-TALK

Postpartum Depression for Moms: 1-800-773-6667

Number for emergency: 911 anywhere in the United States

UNITED KINGDOM

The Samaritans 08457-90-90-90

Childline 0800-1111

Papyrus Hopeline 0870-1704000

Number for emergency: 999 or 112

Suicide Prevention Apps

My3

www.my3app.org

Helps people recognize suicidal warning signs. Asks you to choose 3 close contacts that you feel comfortable reaching out to. It helps you create your own safety plan.

Operation Reach Out

www.4mca.com/suicide_prevention_app

Suicide prevention app that encourages people to reach out for help when they are having suicidal thoughts. It is aimed at preventing suicide among military personnel and veterans. It provides contact with a help centre.

Lifeline Canada, International Association for Suicide Prevention

www.thelifelinecanada.ca

The lifeline app is the National free suicide and prevention and awareness app that offers access and guidance to provide support.

Stay Alive: Grassroots Suicide Prevention

www.prevent-suicide.org.UK

This app is a pocket suicide prevention resource for the UK with information and tools to help stay safe in a crisis. It includes a safety plan.

Jason Foundation: "A Friend Asks"

www.jasonfoundation.com

Tools and resources to help a friend or oneself who may be struggling with suicidal thoughts.

Free Suicide Toolkits and Learning Modules

Toolkit for people who have been impacted by a suicide attempt:

www.mentalhealthcommission.ca

Toolkit for people who have been impacted by a suicide loss:

www.mentalhealthcommission.ca

Preventing Suicide: A Community Engagement Toolkit. Step-by-step guide for communities to engage in suicide prevention activities. In English and Russian:

www.who.int/mental_health/suicide-prevention/community_engagement_toolkit_pilot/en

Free Mental Health Apps

Sandra Kiume of Psych Central has listed the top ten free mental health apps. PsychCentral app also provides up to date mental health information.

MindShift

www.anxietycanada.com/resources/mindshift-cbt

A great tool for anxiety available on iPhone and Android, developed by Anxiety BC at www.anxietycanada.com. It teaches relaxation skills, develops new thinking, and suggests healthy activities. Designed for youth but useful to anyone.

PTSD Coach

www.ptsd.va.gov

Helpful for symptoms of combat-related post-traumatic stress, this trusted military app has been downloaded over 100,000 times for iPhone and Android. Featuring versions in French-Canadian and more.

BellyBio Interactive Breathing

www.apps.apple.com/us/app/bellybio-interactive-breathing/id353763955

Wonderful biofeedback device that monitors your breathing and plays sounds reminiscent of ocean waves when you relax. Great for anxiety and stress. iPhone only.

Positive Activity Jackpot

www.play.google.com/store/apps/details?id=t2.paj&hl=en

A unique augmented reality tool that uses the functionality of a smartphone in an innovative way. Combines a professional behavioral health therapy for depression called pleasant event scheduling (PES) with activities available in the user's location, mapped with GPS. For Android only.

Take a Break! Guided Meditations for Stress Relief

www.apps.apple.com/us/app/take-break-guided-meditations/id453857236

From the excellent developers of relaxation apps at www.meditationoasis.com comes this free app to quickly recharge. Listen to a seven-minute Work Break or 13-minute Stress Relief recording with or without music or nature sounds. iPhone or Android.

Previdence

An assessment tool that allows users to check for symptoms of depression, anxiety, relationship issues, drug and alcohol issues, and other problems and makes recommendations for action. iPhone only.

Operation Reach Out

www.apps.apple.com/ca/app/operation-reach-out/id478899653

This lifesaving app for iPhone and Android was developed by the military to prevent suicide. Recorded videos and menu options help users assess their thinking and reach out for help in crisis.

Relax with Andrew Johnson Lite

www.apps.apple.com/ca/app/relax-andrew-johnson-lite/id307750844

Great guided meditation session for relaxation, helpful with anxiety and stress as well as a sleep aid. Available in Android and iPhone versions.

T2 Mood Tracker

www.apps.apple.com/us/app/t2-mood-tracker/id428373825

Tracks symptoms of depression, anxiety, PTSD, traumatic brain injury, stress and general well-being. Useful to share with clinicians and chart recovery. Another excellent app developed by the Department of Defense National Center for Telehealth and Technology for Android and iPhone.

Relax and Sleep Well with Glenn Harold

www.apps.apple.com/ca/app/relax-sleep-well-by-glenn/id412690467

Twenty-minute guided meditation with music to help you fall asleep. Relaxing and gentle. For iPhone and Android.

Workplace Strategies for Mental Health

The Great-West Life Centre for Mental Health in the Workplace provides free resources to increase workplace mental health knowledge. It provides practical training and tools for employees and managers.

www.workplacestrategiesformentalhealth.com

References

Achor, Shawn, "Discovering Happiness," Calm.com, January 10, 2019

Ackerman, Courtney, "Cognitive Distortions: When Your Brain Lies to You," Positive Psychology Program, Sept 29, 2017

Anderson, Scott, "The Urge to End it All," *The New York Times Magazine*, July 6, 2008

"Are you Feeling Suicidal?" HelpGuide.Org, March 15, 2019

Burkeman, Oliver. "This Column will Change Your Life: Hindsight- it's not just for past events- What were they thinking?" *The Guardian*, April 4, 2019

Centre for Disease Control and Prevention, "Suicide Rising Across the US: More than a mental health concern," June 7, 2018

Cherks, Jason, "The Best Way to Save People from Suicide: What if this is what we should be doing?" *Huffington Post*, November 15, 2018

Cornish, Audie, Host, "Gun Shops Work with Doctors to Prevent Suicide by Firearms," NPR News, November 21, 2018

Deisenhammer, E.A.; Ing, C.M.; Strauss, R., et al, "The Duration of the Suicidal Process: How much time is left for intervention between consideration and accomplishment of a Suicide Attempt?" JClin Psychology, 2009

DeGeneres, Ellen, "Relatable: Netflix Comedy Special," December 18, 2018

Department of National Defense, "Road to Mental Readiness," Mental Health Commission of Canada (2004)

Forbes, Jeremy, "How to Start a Conversation about Suicide," TED Talk, September 15, 2018

Fuller, Kristen, M.D. "5 Common Myths About Suicide Debunked," National Alliance on Mental Illness, September 2018

Galloway, Matt, Host, "Michael Landsberg goes on the record about Mental Health, power of social media, CBC News, November 14, 2017

Gunnell, D., Eddleston, M., Phillips, M.R., Konradsen, F., "The Global Distribution of Fatal Pesticide Self-Poisoning Systematic Review," BMC Public Health, 2007

Hardy, Charlie L., and Van Vugt, "Nice Guys Finish First: The Competitive Altruism Hypothesis," Personality and Social Psychology Bulletin 32, no10 (2006) 1402-13

Harris, Dan, "10% Happier: How I Tamed the Voice in my Head, Reduced Stress Without Losing My Edge, and found Self Help That Actually Works--- A True Story," 2014

Harris, Dan, Host, "10% Happier Podcast. Dr Jennifer Ashton. Life after Suicide," April 3, 2019

Harris, Dan, Host, "10 % Happier Podcast," Anderson Cooper, CNN Anchor, Oct 4, 2017

Harris, Dan. Meditation for Fidgety Skeptics: A 10% Happier How to Book. (2017).

Hartwell, Michael, "Just a Smile Might Save a Life, *Sentinel and Enterprise News*, March 28, 2014

Ilardi, Steve, "Rethinking Depression: Movement is Medicine," Calm.com, April 15, 2019

Inskeep, Steve, Host, "What Happens if You Try and Prevent Every Single Suicide," NPR News, November 2, 2015

Jager-Hyman, S., Cunningham, A., Wenzel, A., et al, "Cognitive Distortions and Suicide Attempts. Cognit Ther Res.," National Center for Biotechnology Information, Aug 1, 2014, 38(4): 369-374

Kelly, Mary Louise, Host, "CDC: US Suicide Rates Have Climbed Dramatically," NPR News, July 7, 2018

King, Noel, Host, "Sharp Increase in Gun Suicides Signals Growing Public Health Crisis," NPR News, July 26, 2018

Klein, Sarah, "10 Things Suicide Attempt Survivors Want You to Know: Learning from the people who have contemplated suicide can help prevent further deaths," Heath.com, July 18, 2018

Kiume, Sandra, Top 10 Free Mental Health Apps, Psych Central:

Knaak, S., Potts, A., Patten, S.B., "Lakeridge Health Opening Minds Evaluation Report," Calgary (AB), Mental Health Commission of Canada; 2012.

Levitin, Dr Daniel, "How to Stay Calm When You Know You'll Be Stressed," TED Talk, October 30, 2015

Levitt, Tamara, "Cognitive Distortions," Calm.com, May 30, 2019

Landsberg, Michael, 'Living with Mental Illness and Addiction," 2015 Conference Keynote Address, Sydney, Nova Scotia

Luxton, D.D., June, J.D., Comtois, K.A., "Can Post Discharge Follow-up Contacts Prevent Suicide and Suicidal Behavior?", National Center for Biotechnology Information, (2013) 34(1) 32-41

Mann, J.J., Apter, A, Bertolote, et al. "Suicide Prevention Strategies A Systemic Review," JAMA 2005, 2064-2074

Mental Health Commission of Canada (MHCC), "Opening Minds Interim Report," Calgary (AB): MHCC; 2013

Miller, Sean, "The Great-West Life Centre for Mental Health in the Workplace," May 9, 2019

Murray, Rheana, "What It is Like to Survive a Suicide Attempt?", Today.com August 3, 2018

Nash, W.P, US Marine Corps and Navy Combat and Operational Stress Continuum Model. A Tool for Leaders in E.C. Ritchie (Ed), Operational Behavioral Health. Washington, D.C: Borden Institute textbook of Military Psychiatry, 2013

Newman, Ed., "A Lesson from 29 Golden Gate Suicide Attempts. Suicide is a Permanent Solution to a Temporary Problem," Medium: Culture, February 20, 2019

Seppala, Emma, "The Happiness Track: How to apply the Science of Happiness to Accelerate Your Success," Harper Collins, 2016

Sinew, Simon, "How Great Leaders Inspire Action: Start with Why," TED Talk, May 25, 2010

"Suicide Prevention Framework: Working Together to Prevent Suicide in Canada – The Federal

Framework for Suicide Prevention," Public Health Agency of Canada, November 24, 2016

Szeto, A., Hamer, A., "Central LHIN Phase 2 Report," Calgary (AB): Mental Health Commission of Canada, 2013

"Telling Your Own Story: Best Practices for Presentations by Suicide Loss and Suicide Attempt Survivors," TheConnectProgram.com, 2018

Timberlake, Justin, "Say Something," Spotify

Tolle, Eckhart, "The Power of Now: A Guide to Spiritual Enlightenment," New World Library, 2004, *O Magazine* 2000 book recommendation

World Health Organization, "Preventing Suicide: A Global Imperative," 2014

Zalsman, G., Hawton, K., Wasserman, D., VanHeeringen, K., Arensman, E., Sarchiapone, M., Purebl, G., "Suicide Prevention Strategies Revealed:10-year Systemic Review, TheLancet.com, (2016) 3(7), 646-659

Zouves, Natasha, "Second Chances: I Survived Jumping off the Golden Gate Bridge," ABC7.com, May 19, 2017

About the Author

Janet MacDonald is a Registered Nurse who has spent over 30 years doing home visits in the community. She is the mother of four adult children and lives in Timberlea, Nova Scotia with her husband Jamie.